Dash Diet Cookbook for Your Dinner

A Mix of recipes perfect to end the day with
taste and stay fit

Natalie Puckett

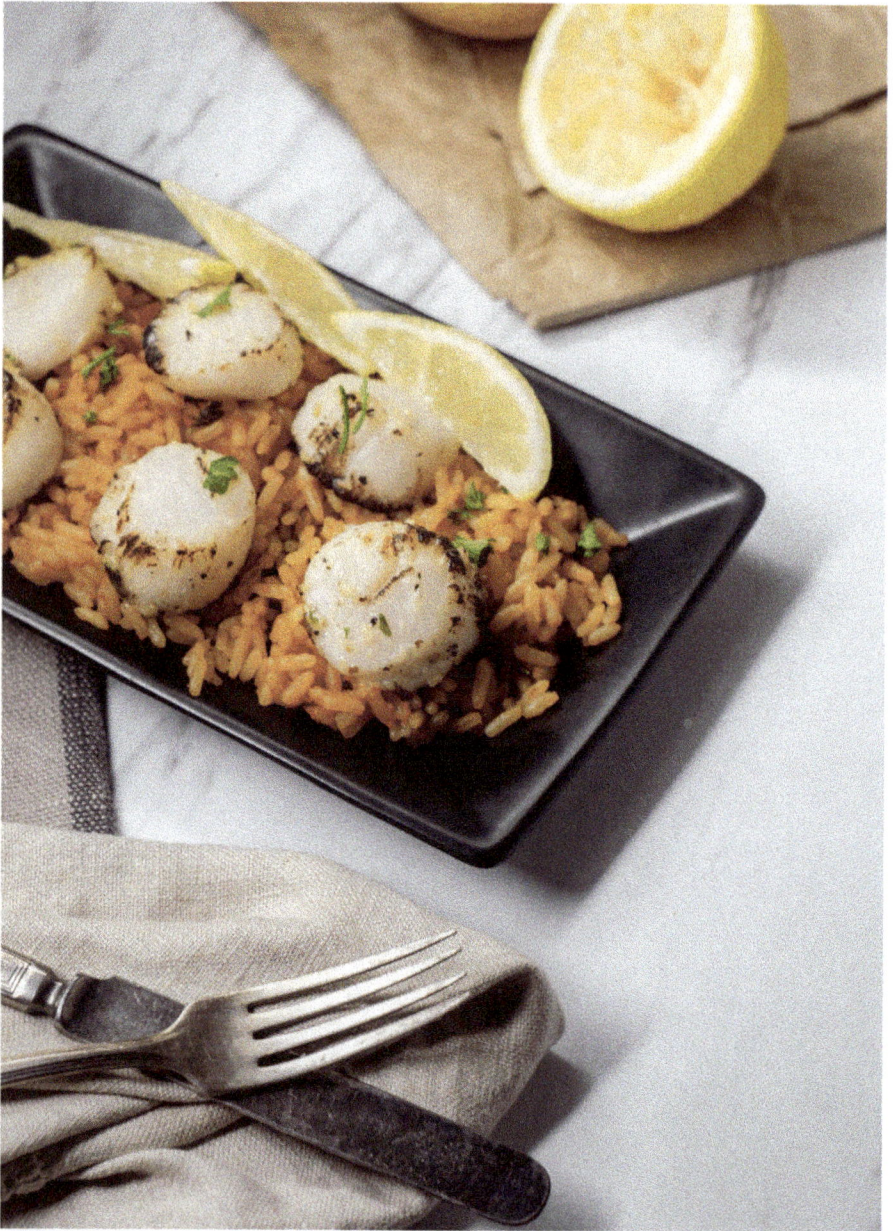

Table of Contents

Lemon and Garlic Scallops

Serving: 4

Prep Time: 10 minutes

Cook Time: 5 minutes

Ingredients:

1 tablespoon olive oil

¼ pounds dried scallops

tablespoons all-purpose flour

¼ teaspoon sunflower seeds

4-5 garlic cloves, minced

1 scallion, chopped

1 pinch of ground sage

lemon juice

tablespoons parsley, chopped

Direction

1. Take a non-stick skillet and place over medium-high heat.

2.   Add oil and permit the oil to heat up.

3.   Take a medium sized bowl and add scallops alongside sunflower seeds and flour.

4.   Place the scallops within the skillet and add scallions, garlic, and sage.

5.   Sauté for 3-4 minutes until they show an opaque texture.

6.   Stir in juice and parsley.

7.   Remove heat and serve hot!

Nutrition (Per Serving)

Calories: 151

Fat: 4g

Carbohydrates: 10g

Protein: 18g

Walnut Encrusted Salmon

Serving: 34

Prep Time: 10 minutes

Cook Time: 14 minutes

Ingredients:

½ cup walnuts

tablespoons stevia

½ tablespoon Dijon mustard

¼ teaspoon dill

salmon fillets (3 ounces each)

1 tablespoon olive oil

Sunflower seeds and pepper to taste

How To:

1.   Pre-heat your oven to 350 degrees F.

2.   Add walnuts, mustard, stevia to kitchen appliance and process until your required consistency is achieved.

3.   Take a frypan and place it over medium heat.

4.   Add oil and let it heat up.

5.   Add salmon and sear for 3 minutes.

6.   Add walnut mix and coat well.

7.   Transfer coated salmon to baking sheet, bake in oven for 8 minutes.

8.   Serve and enjoy!

Nutrition (Per Serving)

Calories: 373

Fat: 43g

Carbohydrates: 4g

Protein: 20g

Roasted Lemon Swordfish

Serving: 4

Prep Time: 10 minutes

Cook Time: 70-80 minutes

Ingredients:

¼ cup parsley, chopped

½ teaspoon garlic, chopped

½ teaspoon canola oil

swordfish fillets, 6 ounces each

¼ teaspoon sunflower seeds

tablespoon sugar

lemons, quartered and seeds removed

How To:

1.   Preheat your oven to 375 degrees F.

2.   Take a small-sized bowl and add sugar, sunflower seeds, lemon wedges.

3.   Toss well to coat them.

4.   Take a shallow baking dish and add lemons, cover with aluminum foil.

5.   Roast for about hour until lemons are tender and browned (Slightly).

6.   Heat your grill and place the rack about 4 inches far away from the source of warmth.

7.   Take a baking pan and coat it with cooking spray.

8.   Transfer fish fillets to the pan and brush with oil on top spread garlic on top.

9.   Grill for about 5 minutes all sides until fillet turns opaque.

10.   Transfer fish to a serving platter, squeeze roasted lemon on top.

11.   Sprinkle parsley, serve with a lemon wedge on the side.

12.   Enjoy!

Nutrition (Per Serving)

Calories: 280

Fat: 12g

Net Carbohydrates: 4g
Protein: 34g

Especial Glazed Salmon

Serving: 4

Prep Time: 45 minutes

Cook Time: 10 minutes

Ingredients:

Pieces of salmon fillets, 5 ounces each

tablespoons coconut aminos

Teaspoon olive oil

2 teaspoons ginger, minced

teaspoons garlic, minced

2 tablespoons sugar-free ketchup

tablespoons dry white wine

2 tablespoons red boat fish sauce, low sodium

How To:

1.   Take a bowl and blend in coconut aminos, garlic, ginger, fish sauce and blend.

2.   Add salmon and let it marinate for 15-20 minutes.

3.   Take a skillet/pan and place it over medium heat.

4.   Add oil and let it heat up.

5.   Add salmon fillets and cook on high heat for 3-4 minutes per side.

6.   Remove dish once crispy.

7.   Add sauce and wine.

8.   Simmer for five minutes on low heat.

9.   Return salmon to the glaze and flip until each side are glazed.

10.   Serve and enjoy!

Nutrition (Per Serving)

Calories: 372

Fat: 24g

Carbohydrates: 3g

Protein: 35g

Generous Stuffed Salmon Avocado

Serving: 2

Prep Time: 10 minutes

Cook Time: 30 minutes

Ingredients:

ripe organic avocado

ounces wild caught smoked salmon

ounce cashew cheese

tablespoons extra virgin olive oil

Sunflower seeds as needed

How To:

1.   Cut avocado in half and deseed.

2.   Add the rest of the ingredients to a food processor and process until coarsely chopped.

3.   Place mixture into avocado.

4.   Serve and enjoy!

Nutrition (Per Serving)

Calories: 525

Fat: 48g

Carbohydrates: 4g

Protein: 19g

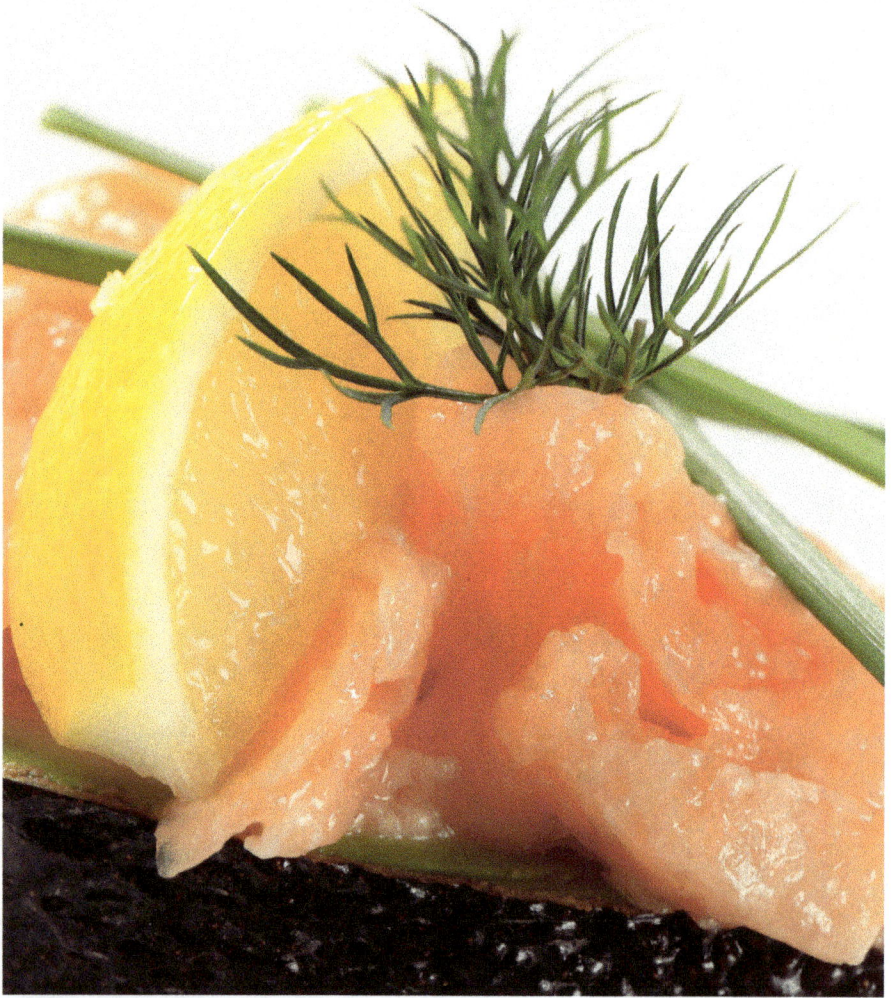

Insalata Capricciosa

Nutrition

Calories: 551 kcal | Gross carbohydrates: 9 g | Protein: 28 g | Fats: 46 g | Fiber: 3 g | Net carbohydrates: 6 g | Macro fats: 58 % | Macro proteins: 35 % | Macro carbohydrates: 8 %

Time: 15 minutes

Ingredients

2 eggs

2 tomatoes around 200 grams

100 grams of mixed lettuce or iceberg lettuce

60 grams of black olives, preferably in olive oil

100 grams of mozzarella

100 grams of tuna in water or olive oil

pepper and salt

50 ml extra virgin olive oil

15 ml of lemon juice

Instructions

1. Bring a saucepan of water to the boil. Once the water boils, carefully lay the eggs in it. Bring the water back to the boil and boil the eggs for 8 minutes. Then place the pan under the cold tap so that the eggs cool sufficiently to allow them to peel.

2.   Wash the tomatoes, pat them dry with kitchen paper and cut into slices.

3.   Drain the tuna well and place it on top of the lettuce.

4.   Also, divide the tomato and olives slices over the lettuce and also cut the boiled eggs into slices. Put it on the lettuce too.

5.   Season the salad with salt and pepper. Make a vinaigrette by mixing the olive oil well with the lemon juice in a cup. Use a teaspoon to distribute the vinaigrette on the plates.

Oopsie sandwich (keto)

Nutrition

Calories: 84 kcal | Gross carbohydrates: 2 g | Protein: 4 g | Fats: 7 g | Fiber: 1g | Net carbohydrates: 1 g | Macro fats: 58 % | Macro proteins: 33 % | Macro carbohydrates: 8 %

Total time: 30 minutes

Ingredients

2 eggs

75 grams of cream cheese

1 teaspoon of psyllium

0.5 teaspoon baking powder

pinch of salt

Instructions

1.   Preheat the oven to 150° Celsius and ensure that the eggs are at room temperature. When the eggs come out of the refrigerator, place them in a bowl of lukewarm tap water for 10-15 minutes.

2.   Split the eggs. Put the egg whites in a cup for a hand blender and the egg yolks in another bowl.

3.   Mix the egg yolks with the cream cheese, the psyllium and the baking powder with a whisk or a fork. Let this batter rest for 5 minutes so that the baking powder and psyllium can work.

4.   Beat the egg whites with a pinch of salt. The proteins must be so stiff that if you hold the cup upside down, they will not move.

5.   Carefully scoop the egg whites through the egg yolk-cream cheese mixture. The mixture must become nicely airy.

6.   Put a sheet of baking paper on an oven plate and make 8 heaps of batter on the baking sheet.

7.   Bake in 25 minutes at 150° Celsius. The sandwiches must be beautifully golden brown.

Keto (gluten-free) poffertjes

Nutrition

Calories: 700 kcal | Gross carbohydrates: 8 g | Protein: 27 g | Fats: 63 g |Fiber: 1 g | Net carbohydrates: 7 g | Macro fats: 65 % | Macro proteins: 28 % |Macro carbohydrates: 7 %

Total time: 40 minutes

Ingredients

Keto poffertjes

4 eggs

250 grams of ricotta

1 tablespoon psyllium, for example, Livinggreens psyllium fibers

0.5 teaspoon baking powder

0.25 teaspoon vanilla extract

2 tablespoons of mild olive oil

Whipped cream

200 ml whipped cream

0.5 teaspoon vanilla extract

Instructions

1.   Allow the eggs to reach room temperature by removing them from the fridge 15 minutes in advance or by placing them in lukewarm tap water for 5 minutes.

2.   If you have made your own ricotta, use a hand blender or hand blender until there are no / few lumps. If you have ricotta from the store this is not necessary.

3.   Now add the ricotta, the baking powder (optional), vanilla extract and the psyllium to the beaten eggs and mix well with a fork.

4.   Let the batter stand for 5-10 minutes so that it becomes a little stronger.

5.   Heat a cast-iron poffertjes pan over high heat so that it becomes hot. Then grease the pan with a mild olive oil with a brush and lower the heat.

6.   Now place a spoonful of batter in each compartment in the pan. Make sure you have lowered the heat now!

7.   Bake the pancake for 2-4 minutes on one side (depending on how large the pancake is). When the top starts to dry, turn the poffertje with a spoon and bake the other side. Repeat until all the batter has been used up.

8.   Beat the whipped cream with the vanilla extract or use a whipped cream machine.

9.   Serve cold or hot.

Notes: Delicious with fresh raspberry or chia raspberry jam or chia blueberry jam or homemade keto-Nutella.

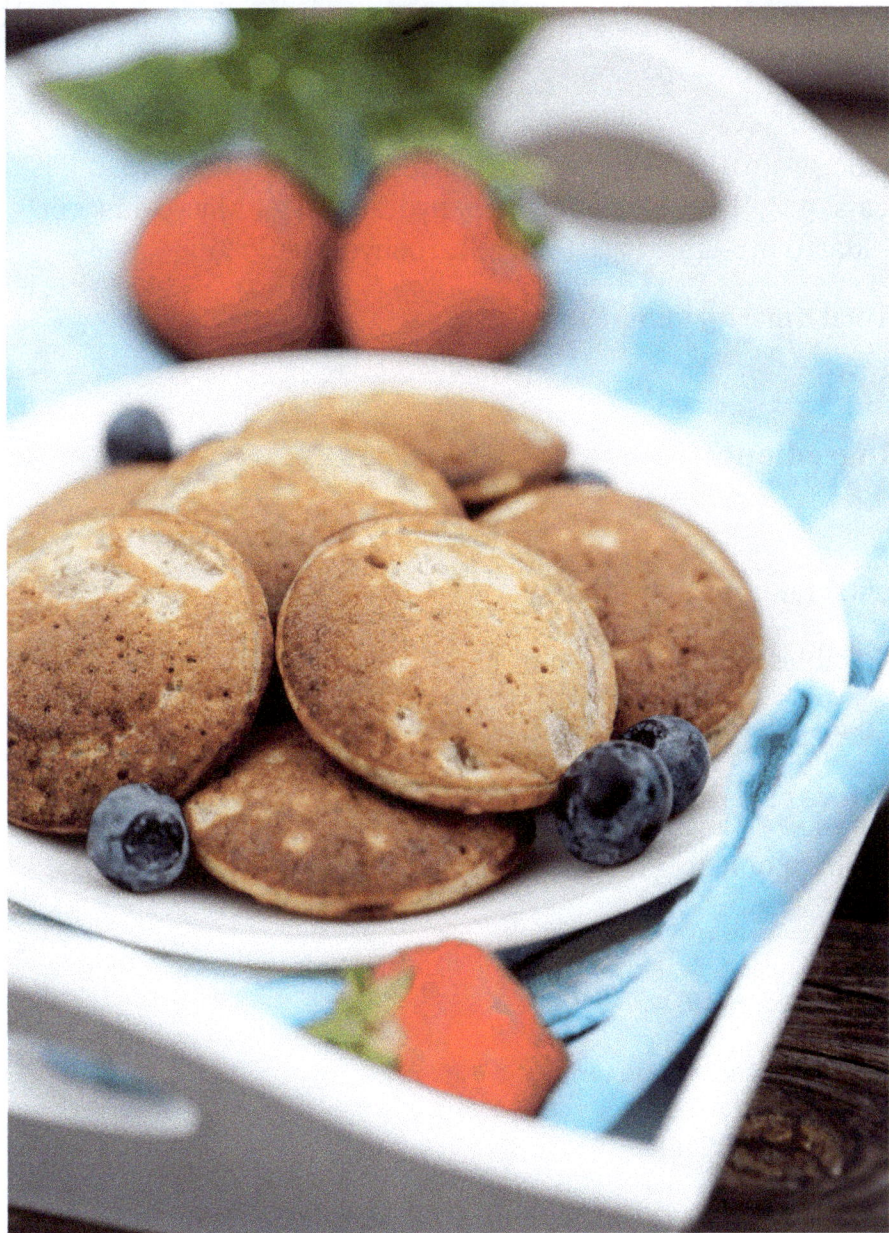

Frittata with Chanterelles

Nutrition

Calories: 1011 kcal | Gross carbohydrates: 13 g | Protein: 21 g | Fats: 97 g |Fiber: 4 g | Net carbohydrates: 9 g | Macro fats: 76 % | Macro proteins: 17 % |Macro carbohydrates: 7 %

Total time: 25 minutes

Ingredients

6 eggs

250 grams of chanterelles

50 tablespoons butter

50 ml extra virgin olive oil

1 clove of garlic

1 tablespoon oregano leaves without stalk

1 tablespoon of young sage leaves

0.5 lemon

300 ml mascarpone

Creme fraiche dip

1 forest outing

200 ml creme fraiche

Instructions

1.   Preheat the oven to 220° Celsius.

2.   If the eggs are not yet at room temperature, remove them from the refrigerator and place them in a bowl of warm water (not boiling!).

3.   Use a mushroom brush to gently clean the chanterelles. Leave them whole.

4.   Heat the butter with the olive oil in a frying pan. Add the chanterelles to the pan as soon as the butter has melted and bake for 3-4 minutes until medium to high heat. Turn over occasionally.

5.   Clean the garlic and chop it into small pieces.

6.   Wash the sage and oregano, pat dry and chop into small pieces.

7.   Add the garlic and spices to the skillet and turn the heat down. Cook for 4-5 minutes. Remove the pan from the heat and squeeze half a lemon over the chanterelles.

8.   Grease a baking dish and / or put a sheet of baking paper in it.

9.   Beat the eggs with the mascarpone in a bowl and add some salt and pepper.

10.   Put the chanterelles in the baking dish and pour the beaten eggs over it. Bake in the oven for 10-15 minutes, until the egg is firm.

11.   You can check whether the frittata is fully cooked by piercing it with a wooden or metal stick. If the skewer comes out clean, the frittata is ready.

12.   Clean a spring onion and cut into rings. Mix through the creme fraiche.

13.   Serve with creme fraiche.

The Refreshing Nutter

Serving: 1

Prep Time: 10 minutes

Ingredients:

1 tablespoon chia seeds

2 cups water

1 ounces Macadamia Nuts

1-2 packets Stevia, optional

1 ounce hazelnut

How To:

1.   Add all the listed ingredients to a blender.

2.   Blend on high until smooth and creamy.

3.   Enjoy your smoothie.

Nutrition (Per Serving)

Calories: 452

Fat: 43g

Carbohydrates: 15g

Protein: 9g

Elegant Cranberry Muffins

Serving: 24 muffins

Prep Time: 10 minutes

Cooking Time: 20 minutes

Ingredients:

2 cups almond flour

2 teaspoons baking soda

¼ cup avocado oil

1 whole egg

¾ cup almond milk

½ cup Erythritol

½ cup apple sauce

Zest of 1 orange

2 teaspoons ground cinnamon

2 cup fresh cranberries

How To:

1. Pre-heat your oven to 350 degrees F.

2. Line muffin tin with paper muffin cups and keep them on the side.

3. Add flour, baking soda and keep it on the side.

4. Take another bowl and whisk in remaining ingredients and add flour, mix well.

5. Pour batter into prepared muffin tin and bake for 20 minutes.

6. Once done, let it cool for 10 minutes.

7. Serve and enjoy!

Nutrition (Per Serving)

Total Carbs: 7g

Fiber: 2g

Protein: 2.3g

Fat: 7g

Apple and Almond Muffins

Serving: 6 muffins

Prep Time: 10 minutes

Cooking Time: 20 minutes

Ingredients:

6 ounces ground almonds

1 teaspoon cinnamon

½ teaspoon baking powder

1 pinch sunflower seed

1 whole egg

1 teaspoon apple cider vinegar

2 tablespoons Erythritol

1/3 cup apple sauce

How To:

1.   Pre-heat your oven to 350 degrees F.

2.   Line muffin tin with paper muffin cups, keep them on the side.

3.   Mix in almonds, cinnamon, baking powder, sunflower seeds and keep it on the side.

4.   Take another bowl and beat in eggs, apple cider vinegar, apple sauce, Erythritol.

5.   Add the mix to dry ingredients and mix well until you have a smooth batter.

6.   Pour batter into tin and bake for 20 minutes.

7.   Once done, let them cool.

8.   Serve and enjoy!

Nutrition (Per Serving)

Total Carbs: 10

Fiber: 4g

Protein: 13g

Fat: 17g

Stylish Chocolate Parfait

Serving: 4

Prep Time: 2 hours

Cook Time: nil

Ingredients:

2 tablespoons cocoa powder

1 cup almond milk

1 tablespoon chia seeds

Pinch of sunflower seeds

½ teaspoon vanilla extract

How To:

1.   Take a bowl and add cocoa powder, almond milk, chia seeds, vanilla extract and stir.

2.   Transfer to dessert glass and place in your fridge for 2 hours.

3.   Serve and enjoy!

Nutrition (Per Serving)

Calories: 130

Fat: 5g

Carbohydrates: 7g

Protein: 16g

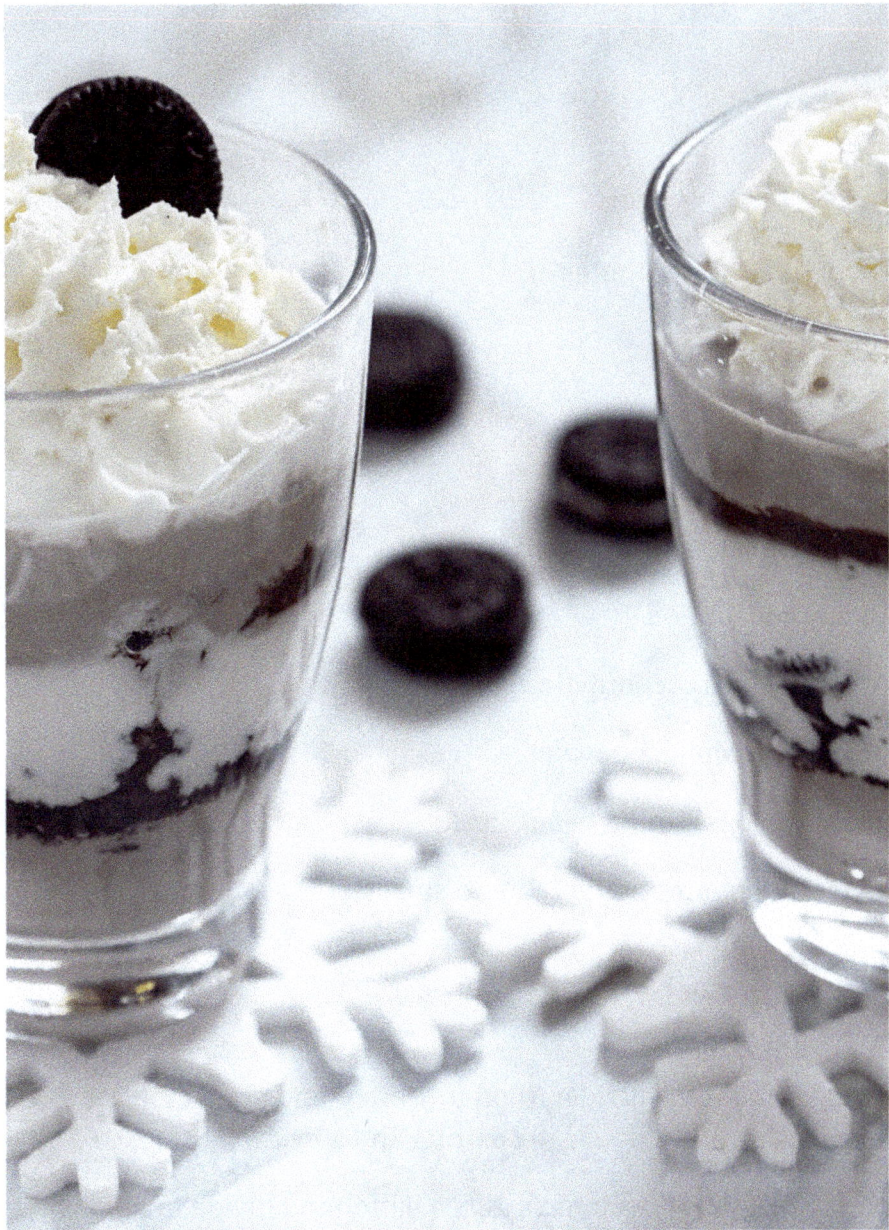

Supreme Matcha Bomb

Serving: 10

Prep Time: 100 minutes

Cook Time: Nil

Ingredients:

3/4 cup hemp seeds

½ cup coconut oil

2 tablespoons coconut almond butter

1 teaspoon Matcha powder

2 tablespoons vanilla bean extract

½ teaspoon mint extract Liquid stevia

How To:

1.   Take your blender/food processor and add hemp seeds, coconut oil, Matcha, vanilla extract and stevia.

2.   Blend until you have a nice batter and divide into silicon molds.

3. Melt coconut almond butter and drizzle on top.

4. Let the cups chill and enjoy!

Nutrition (Per Serving)

Calories: 200

Fat: 20g

Carbohydrates: 3g

Protein: 5g

Mesmerizing Avocado and Chocolate Pudding

Serving: 2

Prep Time: 30 minutes

Cook Time: Nil

Ingredients:

1 avocado, chunked

1 tablespoon natural sweetener such as stevia

2 ounces cream cheese, at room temp

¼ teaspoon vanilla extract

4 tablespoons cocoa powder, unsweetened

How To:

1.   Blend listed ingredients in blender until smooth.

2.   Divide the mix between dessert bowls, chill for 30 minutes.

3.   Serve and enjoy!

Nutrition (Per Serving)

Calories: 281

Fat: 27g

Carbohydrates: 12g

Protein: 8g

Hearty Pineapple Pudding

Serving: 4

Prep Time: 10 minutes

Cooking Time: 5 hours

Ingredients:

1 teaspoon baking powder

1 cup coconut flour

3 tablespoons stevia

3 tablespoons avocado oil

½ cup coconut milk

½ cup pecans, chopped

½ cup pineapple, chopped

½ cup lemon zest, grated

1 cup pineapple juice, natural

How To:

1.   Grease Slow Cooker with oil.

2.   Take a bowl and mix in flour, stevia, baking powder, oil, milk, pecans, pineapple, lemon zest, pineapple juice and stir well.

3.   Pour the mix into the Slow Cooker.

4.   Place lid and cook on LOW for 5 hours.

5.   Divide between bowls and serve.

6.   Enjoy!

Nutrition (Per Serving)

Calories: 188

Fat: 3g

Carbohydrates: 14g

Protein: 5g

The Mean Green Smoothie

Serving: 2

Prep Time: 5 minutes

Ingredients:

1 avocado

1 handful spinach, chopped

Cucumber, 2 inch slices, peeled

1 lime, chopped

Handful of grapes, chopped

5 dates, stoned and chopped

1 cup apple juice (fresh)

How To:

1.   Add all the listed ingredients to your blender.

2.   Blend until smooth.

3.   Add a few ice cubes and serve the smoothie.

4.   Enjoy!

Nutrition (Per Serving)

Calories: 200

Fat: 10g

Carbohydrates: 14g

Protein 2g

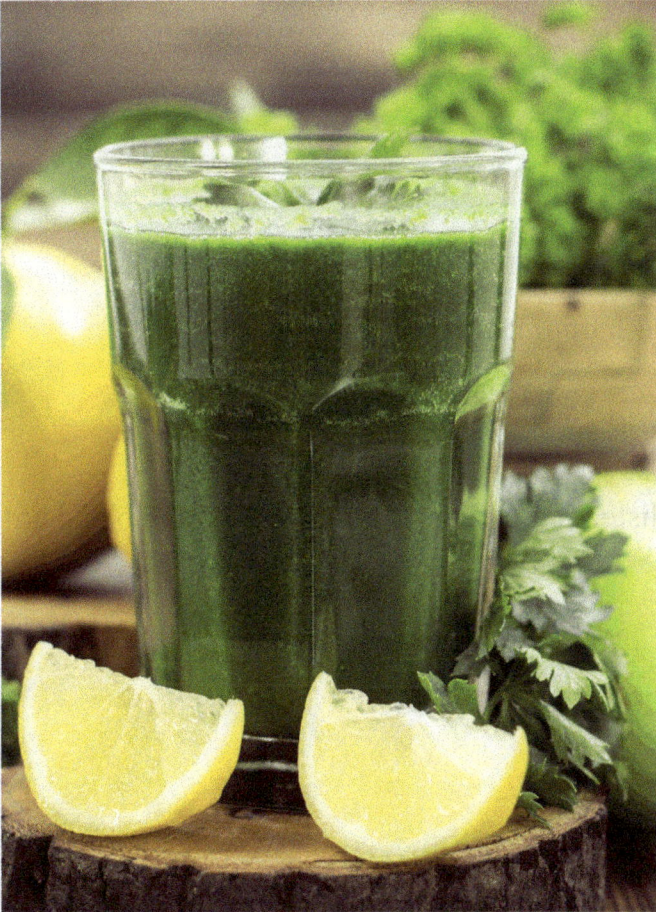

Mint Flavored Pear Smoothie

Serving: 2

Prep Time: 5 minutes

Ingredients:

¼ honey dew

2 green pears, ripe

½ apple, juiced 1 cup ice cubes

½ cup fresh mint leaves

How To:

Add the listed ingredients to your blender and blend until smooth. Serve chilled!

Nutrition (Per Serving)

Calories: 200

Fat: 10g

Carbohydrates: 14g

Protein 2g

Chilled Watermelon Smoothie

Serving: 2

Prep Time: 5 minutes

Ingredients:

1 cup watermelon chunks

½ cup coconut water

1 ½ teaspoons lime juice

4 mint leaves

4 ice cubes

How To:

1.   Add the listed ingredients to your blender and blend until smooth.

2.   Serve chilled!

Nutrition (Per Serving)

Calories: 200

Fat: 10g

Carbohydrates: 14g

Protein 2g

Banana Ginger Medley

Serving: 2

Prep Time: 5 minutes

Ingredients:

1 banana, sliced

¾ cup vanilla yogurt

1 tablespoon honey

½ teaspoon ginger, grated

How To:

1.   Add the listed ingredients to your blender and blend until smooth.

2.   Serve chilled!

Nutrition (Per Serving)

Calories: 200
Fat: 10g
Carbohydrates: 14g
Protein 2g

Banana and Almond Flax Glass

Serving: 2

Prep Time: 5 minutes

Ingredients:

1 ripe frozen banana, diced

2/3 cup unsweetened almond milk

1/3 cup fat free plain Greek Yogurt

1 ½ tablespoons almond butter

1 tablespoon flaxseed meal

1 teaspoon honey

2-3 drops almond extract

How To:

Add the listed ingredients to your blender and blend until smooth

Serve chilled!

Nutrition (Per Serving)

Calories: 200

Fat: 10g

Carbohydrates: 14g

Protein: 2g

Spicy Wasabi Mayonnaise

Serving: 4

Prep Time: 15 minutes

Cook Time: Nil

Ingredients:

1 cup mayonnaise

½ tablespoon wasabi paste

How To:

1. Take a bowl and mix wasabi paste and mayonnaise.

2. Mix well.

3. Let it chill and use as needed.

Nutrition (Per Serving)

Calories: 388

Fat: 42g

Carbohydrates: 1g

Protein: 1g

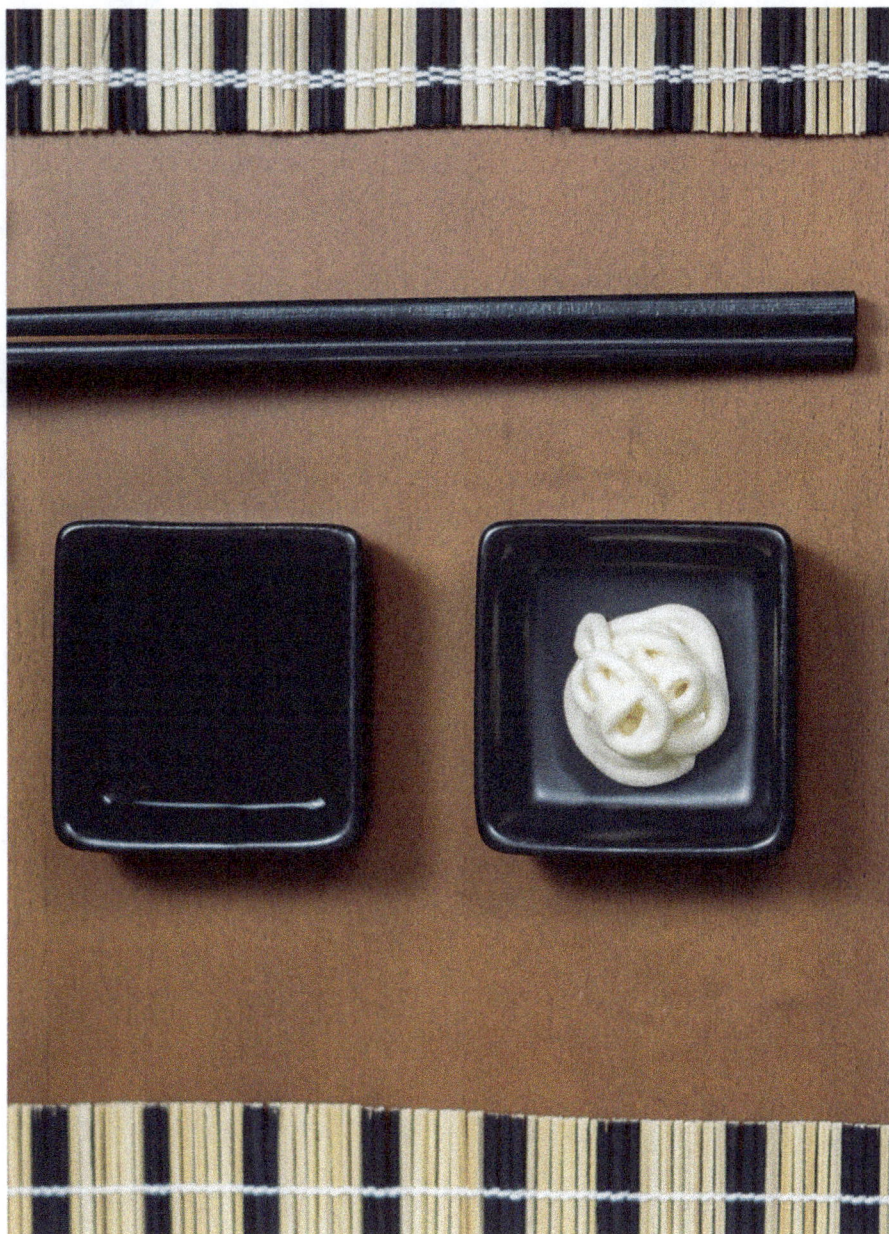

Mediterranean Kale Dish

Serving: 6

Prep Time: 15 minutes

Cook Time: 10 minutes

Ingredients:

12 cups kale, chopped

2 tablespoons lemon juice

1 tablespoon olive oil

1 teaspoon coconut aminos

Sunflower seeds and pepper as needed

How To:

1.   Add a steamer insert to your saucepan.

2.   Fill the saucepan with water up to the bottom of the steamer.

3.   Cover and bring water to boil (medium-high heat).

4.   Add kale to the insert and steam for 7-8 minutes.

5.   Take a large bowl and add lemon juice, olive oil,

sunflower seeds, coconut aminos, and pepper.

6.   Mix well and add the steamed kale to the bowl.

7.   Toss and serve.

8.   Enjoy!

Nutrition (Per Serving)

Calories: 350

Fat: 17g

Carbohydrates: 41g

Protein: 11g

Delicious Garlic Tomatoes

Serving: 4

Prep Time: 10 minutes

Cook Time: 50 minutes

Ingredients:

4 garlic cloves, crushed

1 pound mixed cherry tomatoes

3 thyme sprigs, chopped

Pinch of sunflower seeds

Black pepper as needed

¼ cup olive oil

How To:

1. Preheat your oven to 325 degrees F.
2. Take a baking dish and add tomatoes, olive oil and thyme.
3. Season with sunflower seeds and pepper and mix.
4. Bake for 50 minutes.

5. Divide tomatoes and pan juices and serve.

6. Enjoy!

Nutrition (Per Serving)

Calories: 100

Fat: 0g

Carbohydrates: 1g

Protein: 6g

Mashed Celeriac

Serving: 4

Prep Time: 10 minutes

Cook Time: 20 minutes

Ingredients:

2 celeriac, washed, peeled and diced

2 teaspoons extra-virgin olive oil

1 tablespoon honey

½ teaspoon ground nutmeg

Sunflower seeds and pepper as needed

How To:

1.   Pre-heat your oven to 400 degrees F.

2.   Line a baking sheet with aluminum foil and keep it on the side.

3.   Take a large bowl and toss celeriac and olive oil.

4.   Spread celeriac evenly on a baking sheet.

5.   Roast for 20 minutes until tender.

6.   Transfer to a large bowl.

7.   Add honey and nutmeg.

8.   Use a potato masher to mash the mixture until fluffy.

9.   Season with sunflower seeds and pepper.

10.   Serve and enjoy!

Nutrition (Per Serving)

Calories: 136

Fat: 3g

Carbohydrates: 26g

Protein: 4g

Cool Mushroom Munchies

Serving: 2

Prep Time: 5 minutes

Cook Time: 10 minutes

Ingredients:

4 Portobello mushroom caps

3 tablespoons coconut aminos

2 tablespoons sesame oil

1 tablespoon fresh ginger, minced

1 small garlic clove, minced

How To:

1.   Set your broiler to low, keeping the rack 6 inches from the heating source.

2.   Wash mushrooms under cold water and transfer them to a baking sheet (top side down).

3.   Take a bowl and blend in vegetable oil , garlic, coconut aminos, ginger and pour the mixture over the mushrooms tops .

4.   Cook for 10 minutes.

5.   Serve and enjoy!

Nutrition (Per Serving)

Calories: 196

Fat: 14g

Carbohydrates: 14g

Protein: 7g

Banana and Buckwheat Porridge

Serving: 2

Prep Time: 10 minutes

Cook Time: 15 minutes

Ingredients:

1 cup of water

1 cup buckwheat groats

2 big grapefruits, peeled and sliced

1 tablespoon ground cinnamon

3-4 cups almond milk

2 tablespoons natural almond butter

How To:

1.   Take a medium-sized saucepan and add buckwheat and water.

2.   Place the pan over medium heat and convey to a boil.

3.   Keep cooking until the buckwheat absorbs the water.

4.   Reduce heat to low and add almond milk, stir gently.

5. Add the remainder of the ingredients (except the grapefruits).

6. Stir and take away from the warmth.

7. Transfer into cereal bowls and add grapefruit chunks.

8. Serve and enjoy!

Nutrition (Per Serving)

Calories: 223

Fat: 4g

Carbohydrates: 4g

Protein: 7g

Delightful Berry Quinoa Bowl

Serving: 4

Prep Time: 5 minutes

Cook Time: 15 minutes

Ingredients:

1 cup quinoa

2 cups of water

1 piece, 2-inch sized cinnamon stick

2-3 tablespoons of maple syrup

Flavorful Toppings

½ cup blueberries, raspberries or strawberries

2 tablespoons raisins

1 teaspoon lime

¼ teaspoon nutmeg, grated

3 tablespoons whipped coconut cream

2 tablespoon cashew nuts, chopped

How To:

1.   Take a metal strainer and pass your grain through them to strain them well.

2.   Rinse the grains under cold water thoroughly.

3.   Take a medium-sized saucepan and pour within the water.

4.   Add the strained grains and convey the entire mixture to a boil.

5.   Add cinnamon sticks and canopy the saucepan.

6.   Lower the warmth and let the mixture simmer for quarter-hour to permit the grain to soak up the liquid.

7.   Remove the warmth and plump up the mixture employing a fork.

8.   Add syrup if you would like additional flavor.

9.   Also, if you're looking to form things a touch more interesting, just add any of the abovementioned ingredients.

Nutrition (Per Serving)

Calories: 202

Fat: 5g

Carbohydrates: 35g

Protein: 6g

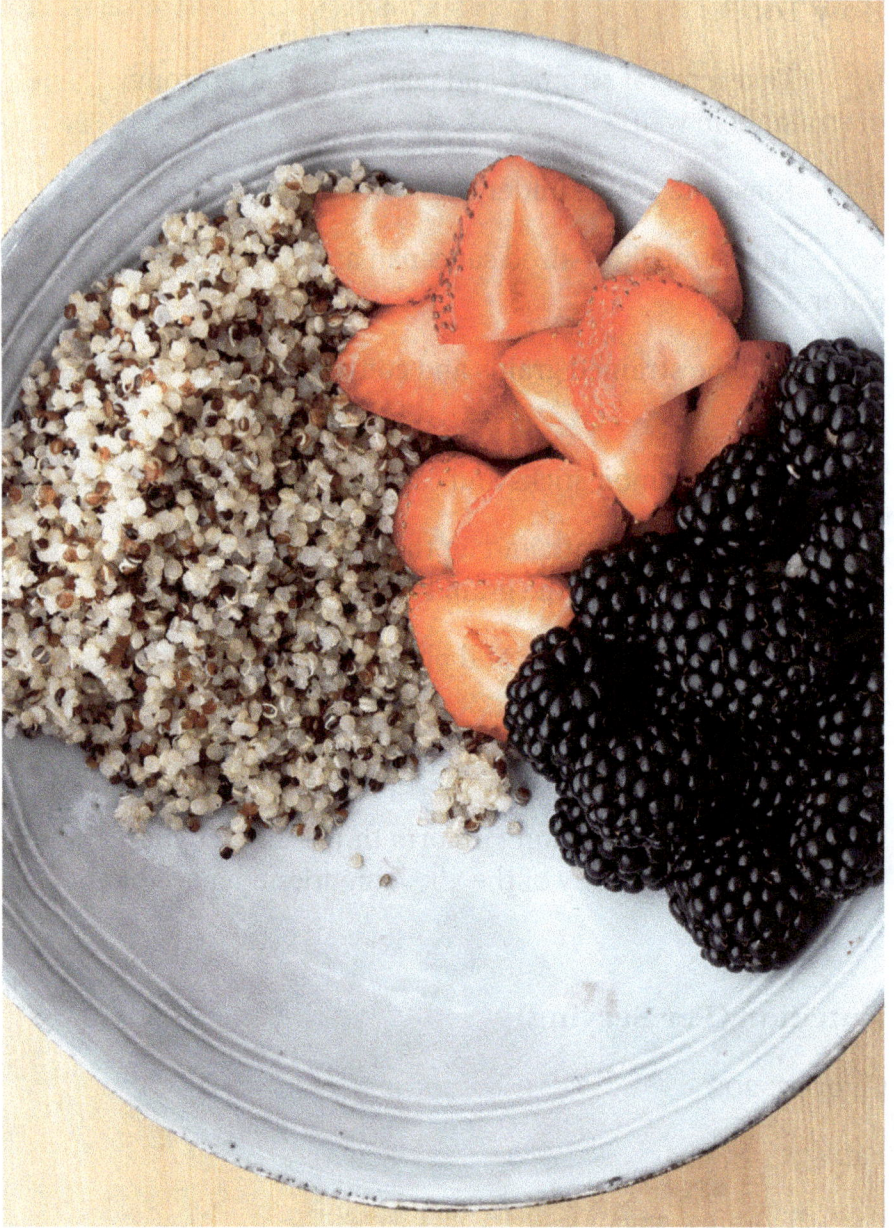

Fantastic Bowl of Steel Oats

Serving: 4

Prep Time: 5 minutes

Cook Time: 25 minutes

Ingredients:

3 ¾ cup water

1 ¼ cup steel-cut oats

¼ teaspoon salt

Flavorful Toppings

1 teaspoon cinnamon

½ teaspoon nutmeg

½ teaspoon lemon pepper

1 teaspoon Garam masala

Mixed berries as needed

Diced mangos as needed

Sliced bananas as needed

Dried fruits as needed

Nuts as needed

Flavorful Toppings

1 tablespoon coconut milk

How To:

1.   Take a medium-sized saucepan and convey it over high heat.

2.   Add water and permit the water to heat up.

3.   Add the steel-cut oats with some salt and lower the warmth to medium-low.

4.   Let the mixture simmer for about 25 minutes, ensuring to stay stirring it all the way.

5.   Add coconut milk or almond butter for a few extra flavor.

6.   Once done, serve with some berries or nuts.

7.   Enjoy!

Nutrition (Per Serving)

Calories: 125

Fat: 3g

Carbohydrates: 20g

Protein: 7g

Quinoa and Cinnamon Bowl

Serving: 2

Prep Time: 10 minutes

Cook Time: 15 minutes

Ingredients:

1 cup uncooked quinoa

1½ cups water

½ teaspoon ground cinnamon

½ teaspoon sunflower seeds

A drizzle of almond/coconut milk for serving

How To:

1.   Rinse quinoa thoroughly underwater.

2.   Take a medium-sized saucepan and add quinoa, water, cinnamon, and seeds.

3.   Stir and place it over medium-high heat.

4.   Bring the combination to a boil.

5.   Reduce heat to low and simmer for 10 minutes.

6.   Once cooked, remove from the warmth and let it cool.

7.   Serve with a drizzle of almond or coconut milk.

8.   Enjoy!

Nutrition (Per Serving)

Calories: 255

Fat: 13g

Carbohydrates: 33g

Protein: 5g

Awesome Breakfast Parfait

Serving: 2

Prep Time: 5 minutes

Cook Time: Nil

Ingredients:

1 teaspoon sunflower seeds

½ cup low-fat milk

1 cup all-purpose flour

1 teaspoon vanilla

3 eggs, beaten

1 teaspoon baking soda

2 cups non-fat Greek yogurt

How To:

1.   Hack pretzels into small-sized portions and slice the strawberries.

2.   Add yogurt to rock bottom of the glass and top with pretzel pieces and strawberries.

3.   Add more yogurt and keep repeating until you've got spent all the ingredients.

4.   Enjoy!

Nutrition (Per Serving)

Calorie: 304

Fat: 1g

Carbohydrates: 58g

Protein: 15g

Golden Eggplant Fries

Serving: 8

Prep Time: 10 minutes

Cook Time: 15 minutes

Ingredients:

2 eggs

2 cups almond flour

2 tablespoons coconut oil, spray

2 eggplant, peeled and cut thinly Sunflower seeds and pepper

How To:

1.   Preheat your oven to 400 degrees F.

2.   Take a bowl and blend with sunflower seeds and black pepper.

3.   Take another bowl and beat eggs until frothy.

4.   Dip the eggplant pieces into the eggs.

5.   Then coat them with the flour mixture.

6.   Add another layer of flour and egg.

7.   Then, take a baking sheet and grease with copra oil on top.

8.   Bake for about quarter-hour.

9.   Serve and enjoy!

Nutrition (Per Serving)

Calories: 212

Fat: 15.8g

Carbohydrates: 12.1g

Protein: 8.6g

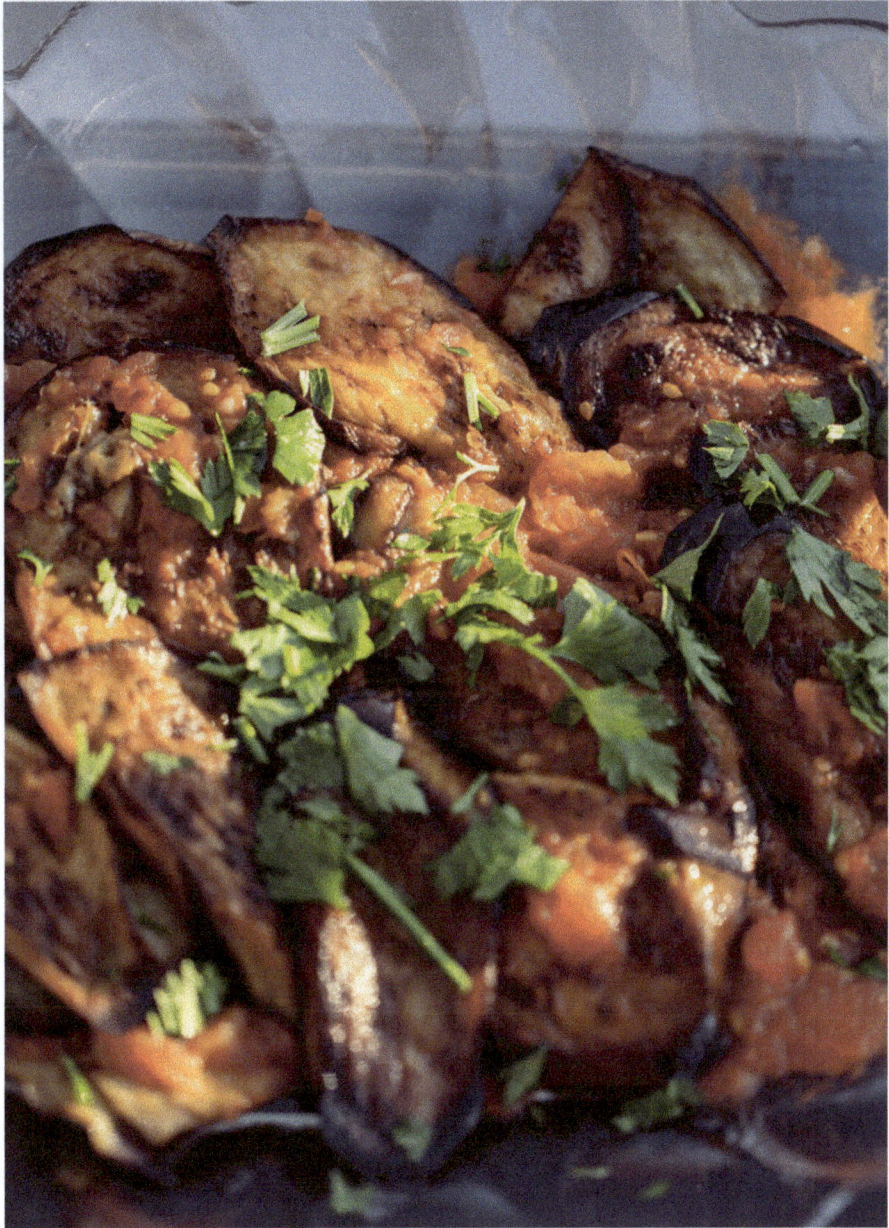

Traditional Black Bean Chili

Serving: 4

Prep Time: 10 minutes

Cooking Time: 4 hours

Ingredients:

1 ½ cups red bell pepper, chopped

1 cup yellow onion, chopped

1 ½ cups mushrooms, sliced

1 tablespoon olive oil

1 tablespoon chili powder

2 garlic cloves, minced

1 teaspoon chipotle chili pepper, chopped ½ teaspoon cumin, ground

16 ounces canned black beans, drained and rinsed

2 tablespoons cilantro, chopped

1 cup tomatoes, chopped

How To:

1.   Add red bell peppers, onion, dill, mushrooms, flavor, garlic, chili pepper, cumin, black beans, tomatoes to your Slow Cooker.

2.   Stir well.

3.   Place lid and cook on HIGH for 4 hours.

4.   Sprinkle cilantro on top.

5.   Serve and enjoy!

Nutrition (Per Serving)

Calories: 211

Fat: 3g

Carbohydrates: 22g

Protein: 5g

Very Wild Mushroom Pilaf

Serving: 4

Prep Time: 10 minutes

Cooking Time: 3 hours

Ingredients:

1 cup wild rice

2 garlic cloves, minced

6 green onions, chopped

2 tablespoons olive oil

½ pound baby Bella mushrooms

2 cups water

How To:

1.   Add rice, garlic, onion, oil, mushrooms and water to your Slow Cooker.

2.   Stir well until mixed.

3.   Place lid and cook on LOW for 3 hours.

4.	Stir pilaf and divide between serving platters.

5.	Enjoy!

Nutrition (Per Serving)

Calories: 210

Fat: 7g

Carbohydrates: 16g

Protein: 4g

Green Palak Paneer

Serving: 4

Prep Time: 5 minutes

Cook Time: 10 minutes

Ingredients:

1-pound spinach

2 cups cubed paneer (vegan)

2 tablespoons coconut oil

1 teaspoon cumin

1 chopped up onion

1-2 teaspoons hot green chili minced up

1 teaspoon minced garlic

15 cashews

4 tablespoons almond milk

1 teaspoon Garam masala

Flavored vinegar as needed

How To:

1.   Add cashews and milk to a blender and blend well.

2.   Set your pot to Sauté mode and add coconut oil; allow the oil to heat up.

3.   Add cumin seeds, garlic, green chilies, ginger and sauté for 1 minute.

4.   Add onion and sauté for two minutes.

5.   Add chopped spinach, flavored vinegar and a cup of water.

6.   Lock up the lid and cook on high for 10 minutes.

7.   Quick-release the pressure.

8.   Add ½ cup of water and blend to a paste.

9.   Add cashew paste, paneer and Garam Masala and stir thoroughly.

10.   Serve over hot rice!

Nutrition (Per Serving)

Calories: 367
Fat: 26g
Carbohydrates: 21g
Protein: 16g

Sporty Baby Carrots

Serving: 4

Prep Time: 5 minutes

Cook Time: 5 minutes

Ingredients:

1-pound baby carrots

1 cup water

1 tablespoon clarified ghee

1 tablespoon chopped up fresh mint leaves Sea flavored vinegar as needed

How To:

1.   Place a steamer rack on top of your pot and add the carrots.

2.   Add water.

3.   Lock the lid and cook at high for two minutes.

4.   Do a fast release.

5.   Pass the carrots through a strainer and drain them.

6.   Wipe the insert clean.

7. Return the insert to the pot and set the pot to Sauté mode.

8. Add drawn butter and permit it to melt.

9. Add mint and sauté for 30 seconds.

10. Add carrots to the insert and sauté well.

11. Remove them and sprinkle with little bit of flavored vinegar on top.

12. Enjoy!

Nutrition (Per Serving)

Calories: 131

Fat: 10g

Carbohydrates: 11g

Protein: 1g

Almond Butter Pork Chops

Serving: 2

Prep Time: 5 minutes

Cook Time: 25 minutes

Ingredients:

1 tablespoon almond butter, divided

2 boneless pork chops

Pepper to taste

1 tablespoon dried Italian seasoning, low fat and low sodium

1 tablespoon olive oil

How To:

1. Pre-heat your oven to 350 degrees F.

2. Pat pork chops dry with a towel and place them during a baking dish.

3. Season with pepper, and Italian seasoning.

4. Drizzle vegetable oil over pork chops.

5. Top each chop with ½ tablespoon almond butter.

6.   Bake for 25 minutes.

7.   Transfer pork chops on two plates and top with almond butter juice.

8.   Serve and enjoy!

Nutrition (Per Serving)

Calories: 333

Fat: 23g

Carbohydrates: 1g

Protein: 31g

Chicken Salsa

Serving: 1

Prep Time: 4 minutes

Cook Time: 14 minutes

Ingredients:

2 chicken breasts

1 cup salsa

1 taco seasoning mix

1 cup plain Greek Yogurt

½ cup of kite ricottta/cashew cheese, cubed

How To:

1.   Take a skillet and place over medium heat.

2.   Add pigeon breast, ½ cup of salsa and taco seasoning.

3.   Mix well and cook for 12-15 minutes until the chicken is completed.

4.   Take the back off and cube them.

5.   Place the cubes on toothpick and top with cheddar.

6.   Place yogurt and remaining salsa in cups and use as dips.

7. Enjoy!

Nutrition (Per Serving)

Calories: 359

Fat: 14g

Net Carbohydrates: 14g

Protein: 43g

Healthy Mediterranean Lamb Chops

Serving: 4

Prep Time: 10 minutes

Cook Time: 10 minutes

Ingredients:

4 lamb shoulder chops, 8 ounces each

2 tablespoons Dijon mustard

2 tablespoons Balsamic vinegar

½ cup olive oil

2 tablespoons shredded fresh basil

How To:

1.   Pat your lamb chop dry employing a kitchen towel and arrange them on a shallow glass baking dish.

2.   Take a bowl and a whisk in Dijon mustard, balsamic vinegar, pepper and blend them well.

3.   Whisk within the oil very slowly into the marinade until the mixture is smooth

4.   Stir in basil.

5.   Pour the marinade over the lamb chops and stir to coat each side well.

6.   Cover the chops and permit them to marinate for 1-4 hours (chilled).

7.   Take the chops out and leave them for half-hour to permit the temperature to succeed in a traditional level.

8.   Pre-heat your grill to medium heat and add oil to the grate.

9.   Grill the lamb chops for 5-10 minutes per side until each side are browned.

10.   Once the middle reads 145 degrees F, the chops are ready, serve and enjoy!

Nutrition (Per Serving)

Calories: 521

Fat: 45g

Carbohydrates: 3.5g

Protein: 22g

Amazing Sesame Breadsticks

Serving: 5 breadsticks

Prep Time: 10 minutes

Cooking Time: 20 minutes

Ingredients:

1 egg white

2 tablespoons almond flour

1 teaspoon Himalayan pink sunflower seeds

1 tablespoon extra-virgin olive oil

½ teaspoon sesame seeds

How To:

1.   Pre-heat your oven to 320 degrees F.

2.   Line a baking sheet with parchment paper and keep it on the side.

3.   Take a bowl and whisk in egg whites, add flour and half sunflower seeds and vegetable oil.

4.   Knead until you've got a smooth dough.

5.   Divide into 4 pieces and roll into breadsticks.

6.   Place on prepared sheet and brush with vegetable oil , sprinkle sesame seeds and remaining sunflower seeds.

7.   Bake for 20 minutes.

8.   Serve and enjoy!

Nutrition (Per Serving)

Total Carbs: 1.1g

Fiber: 1g

Protein: 1.6g

Fat: 5g

Cucumber and Zucchini Soup

Serving: 3

Prep Time: 10 minutes + Chill time

Cook Time: nil

Ingredients:

2 tablespoons olive oil

1 tablespoon fresh dill

2/5 cup fresh cream

7 ounces cucumber, cubed

10 ½ zucchini, cubed

1 red pepper, chopped

3 celery stalks, chopped

Sunflower seeds and pepper to taste

How To:

1.   Add all the veggies during a juice and make a smooth juice.

2.   Mix within the fresh cream and vegetable oil.

3. Season with pepper and sunflower seeds.

4. Garnish with dill.

5. Serve chilled and enjoy!

Nutrition (Per Serving)

Calories: 100

Fat: 8g

Carbohydrates: 4g

Protein: 2g

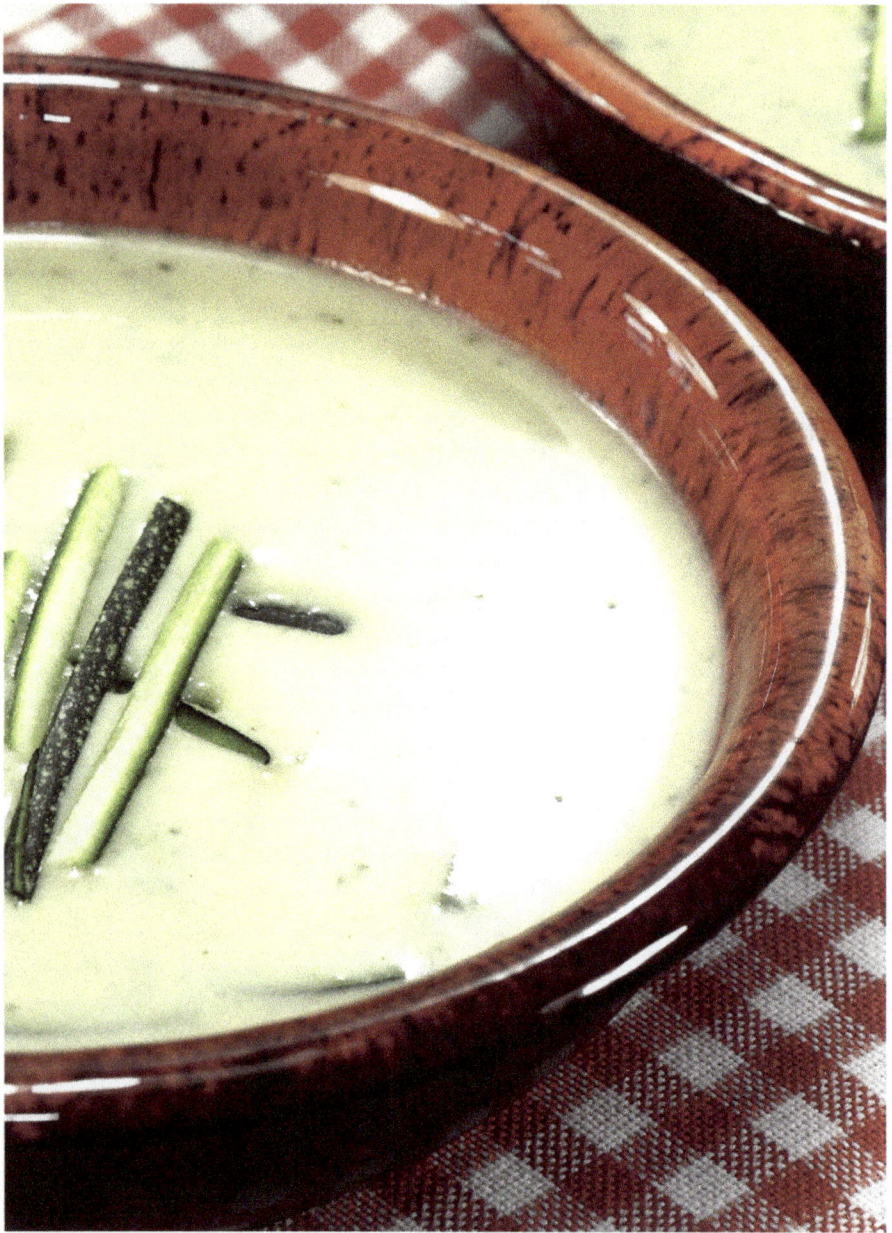

Crockpot Pumpkin Soup

Serving: 3

Prep Time: 10 minutes

Cook Time: 6-8 hours

Ingredients:

1 small pumpkin, halved, peeled, seeds removed, and pulp cubed

2 cups chicken broth

1 cup of coconut almond milk

Sunflower seeds, pepper, thyme, and pepper, to taste

How To:

1.   Add all the ingredients to a crockpot.

2.   Close the lid.

3.   Cook for 6-8 hours on LOW.

4.   Make a smooth puree by employing a blender.

5.   Garnish with roasted seeds.

6.   Serve and enjoy!

Nutrition (Per Serving)

Calories: 60

Fat: 5g

Carbohydrates: 4g

Protein: 4g

Tomato Soup

Serving: 3

Prep Time: 10 minutes

Cook Time: 6-8 hours

Ingredients:

4 cups water or vegetable broth

7 large tomatoes, ripe

½ cup macadamia nuts, raw

1 medium onion, chopped

Sunflower seeds and pepper to taste

How To:

1. Take a nonstick skillet and add the onion.

2. Brown the onion for five minutes.

3. Add all the ingredients to a crockpot.

4. Cook for 6-8 hours on LOW.

5. Make a smooth puree by employing a blender.

6. Serve it warm and enjoy!

Nutrition (Per Serving)

Calories: 145

Fat: 12g

Carbohydrates: 8g

Protein: 6g

Pumpkin, Coconut and Sage Soup

Serving: 3

Prep Time: 10 minutes

Cook Time: 30 minutes

Ingredients:

1 cup pumpkin, canned

6 cups chicken broth

1 cup low fat coconut almond milk

1 teaspoon sage, chopped

3 garlic cloves, peeled

Sunflower seeds and pepper to taste

How To:

1.   Take a stockpot and add all the ingredients except coconut almond milk into it.

2.   Place stockpot over medium heat.

3.   Let it bring back a boil.

4.   Reduce heat to simmer for half-hour.

5.   Add the coconut almond milk and stir.

6.   Serve bacon and enjoy!

Nutrition (Per Serving)

Calories: 145

Fat: 12g

Carbohydrates: 8g

Protein: 6g

Sweet Potato and Leek Soup

Serving: 6

Prep Time: 10 minutes

Cook Time: 8 hours

Ingredients:

6 cups sweet potatoes, peeled and cubed

2 leeks, whites and greens, sliced

6 cups vegetable stock

1 teaspoon dried thyme

1 teaspoon salt

¼ teaspoon fresh ground black pepper

How To:

1.   Add sweet potatoes, leeks, thyme, stock, salt and pepper to your Slow Cooker.

2.   Close lid and cook on LOW for 8 hours.

3.   Mash with potato masher/ use an immersion blender to smooth the soup.

4.   Serve and enjoy!

Nutrition (Per Serving)

Calories: 234

Fat: 2g

Carbohydrates: 47g

Protein: 8g

The Kale and Spinach Soup

Serving: 4

Prep Time: 5 minutes

Cook Time: 10 minutes

Ingredients:

3 ounces coconut oil

8 ounces kale, chopped

2 avocados, diced

4 1/3 cups coconut almond milk

Sunflower seeds and pepper to taste

How To:

1.   Take a skillet and place it over medium heat. 2. Add kale and sauté for 2-3 minutes

2.   Add kale to blender.

3.   Add water, spices, coconut almond milk and avocado to blender also.

4.   Blend until smooth and pour mix into bowl.

5.   Serve and enjoy!

Nutrition (Per Serving)

Calories: 124

Fat: 13g

Carbohydrates: 7g

Protein: 4.2g

Japanese Onion Soup

Serving: 4

Prep Time: 15 minutes

Cook Time: 45 minutes

Ingredients:

½ stalk celery, diced

1 small onion, diced

½ carrot, diced

1 teaspoon fresh ginger root, grated

¼ teaspoon fresh garlic, minced

2 tablespoons chicken stock

3 teaspoons beef bouillon granules

1 cup fresh shiitake, mushrooms

2 quarts water

1 cup baby Portobello mushrooms, sliced

1 tablespoon fresh chives

How To:

1.   Take a saucepan and place it over high heat, add water, bring back a boil.

2.   Add beef bouillon, celery, onion, chicken broth, carrots, half the mushrooms, ginger, garlic.

3.   placed on the lid and reduce heat to medium, cook for 45 minutes.

4.   Take another saucepan and add another half mushroom.

5.   Once the soup is cooked, strain the soup into the pot with uncooked mushrooms.

6.   Garnish with chives and enjoy!

Nutrition (Per Serving)

Calories: 25

Fat: 0.2g

Carbohydrates: 5g

Protein: 1.4g

Amazing Broccoli and Cauliflower Soup

Serving: 4

Prep Time: 10 minutes

Cooking Time: 8 hours

Ingredients:

3 cups broccoli florets

2 cups cauliflower florets

2 garlic cloves, minced

½ cup shallots, chopped

1 carrot, chopped

3 ½ cups low sodium veggie stick

Pinch of pepper

1 cup fat-free milk

6 ounces low-fat cheddar, shredded

1 cup non-fat Greek yogurt

How To:

1.   Add broccoli, cauliflower, garlic, shallots, carrot, stock, pepper to your Slow Cooker.

2.   Stir well and place lid.

3.   Cook on LOW for 8 hours.

4.   Add milk and cheese.

5.   Use an immersion blender to smooth the soup.

6.   Add yogurt and blend another time.

7.   Ladle into bowls and enjoy!

Nutrition (Per Serving)

Calories: 218

Fat: 11g

Carbohydrates: 15g

Protein: 12g

Amazing Zucchini Soup

Serving: 4

Prep Time: 10 minutes

Cook Time: 20 minutes

Ingredients:

1 onion, chopped

3 zucchini, cut into medium chunks

2 tablespoons coconut milk

2 garlic cloves, minced

4 cups chicken stock

2 tablespoons coconut oil

Pinch of salt

Black pepper to taste

How To:

1.   Take a pot and place over medium heat.

2.   Add oil and let it heat up.

3.　　　Add zucchini, garlic, onion and stir.

4.　　　Cook for five minutes.

5.　　　Add stock, salt, pepper and stir.

6.　　　bring back a boil and reduce the warmth.

7.　　　Simmer for 20 minutes.

8.　　　Remove from heat and add coconut milk.

9.　　　Use an immersion blender until smooth.

10.　　Ladle into soup bowls and serve.

11.　　Enjoy!

Nutrition (Per Serving)

Calories: 160

Fat: 2g

Carbohydrates: 4g

Protein: 7g

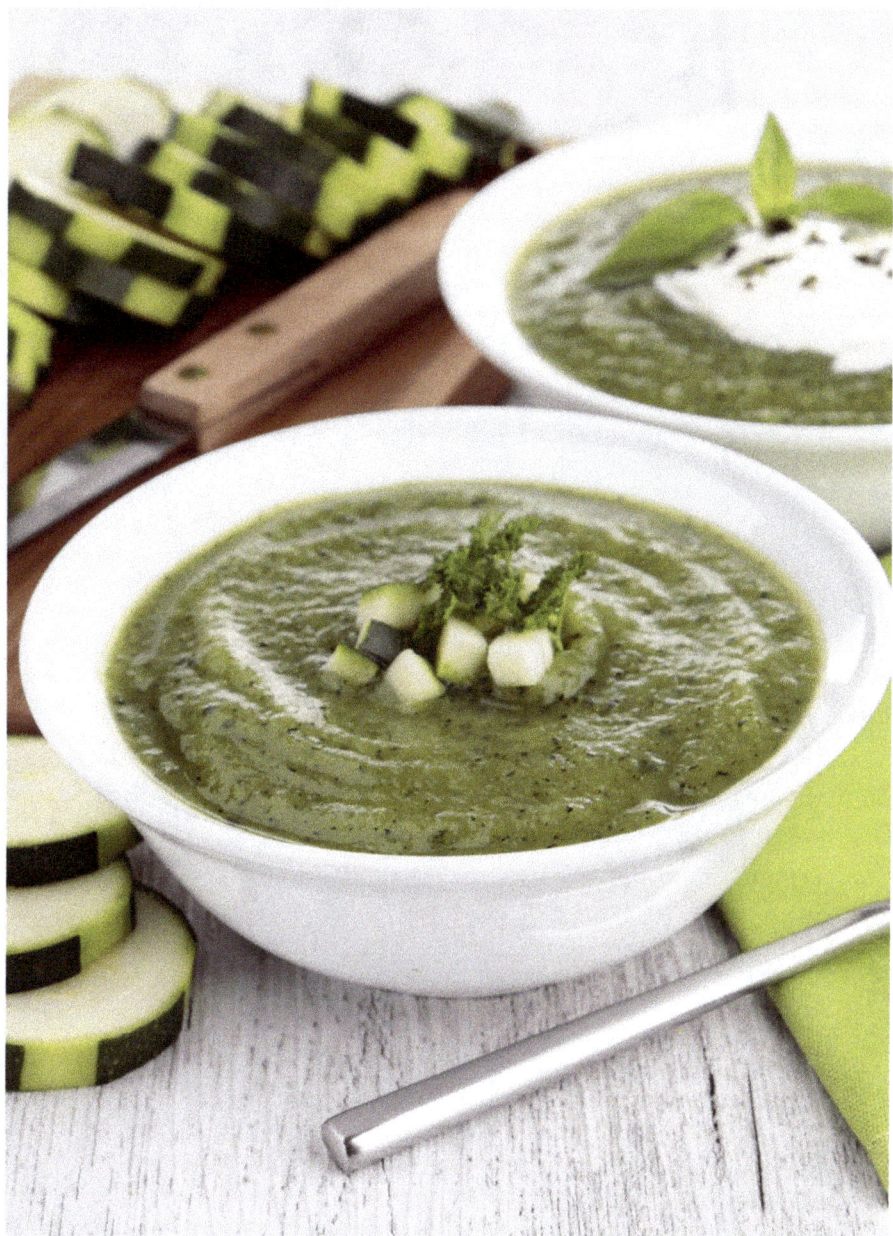

www.ingramcontent.com/pod-product-compliance
Lightning Source LLC
Chambersburg PA
CBHW050750030426
42336CB00012B/1754